Playing the Prescription Game to WIN!

How a middle-class caregiver slashed her husband's monthly drug bill from $538 to $179

By Donna StClair

To Bruce--

"I'm with you 'til the world stops turning,
'Til the end of time--I'm with you."

-- Mickey Jupp; sung by Delbert McClinton

TABLE OF CONTENTS

FOREWORD

I have come to know Donna StClair very well during the time that her husband has been a participant at the Adult Care Center of Central Virginia. From our first meeting, I noticed immediately how well read she was on the subject of his illness, and how she was willing to do whatever it takes to make his life even just a little better. Donna has truly taken her role as "caregiver" to the next level. So, I was not particularly surprised when I learned that she realized one of his needed medications was available from another source for a significantly lower price than what she had paid through his insurance company.

I also was not particularly surprised to learn that she wanted to share her findings with others who are walking in her shoes. Almost every week, I meet with caregivers and family members who are struggling to make ends meet. In all probability, they are paying too much for at least some of their medications, simply because they do not know the right questions to ask or the right places to shop.

Donna has graciously agreed to donate all proceeds from this book to the Adult Care Center of Central Virginia. That doesn't surprise me, either.

--*Kathleen Cresson, RN; Certified Care Manager; Certified Dementia Practitioner;*
Health Care Manager at the Adult Care Center of Central Virginia

PREFACE

I am writing this because I want you to benefit from my mistakes. Otherwise, I have walked a tough path without purpose or legacy. You see, I am going to lose the husband I loved so much to one of dementia's deadly forms, most likely Lewy Body Dementia--the horrendous malady that plagued the late comedian Robin Williams. I may lose myself in the process; the latest statistics indicate that almost half of dementia caregivers die before the person they are trying to care for. Even if I survive, a chunk of me is already gone. Ask any of my friends. and they will tell you that the Donna of today hardly resembles her former self.

For more than 35 years, I lived a fairytale life with my Prince Charming. He was by my side as we hiked, danced, scuba-dived, traveled, antique hunted, attended music concerts, entertained friends. As we inched toward retirement, we were anticipating a life of travels to our beloved National Parks, long hikes along the Appalachian Trail, and evenings of memories, music, wine, and romance.

It would have been so wonderful. If only our personal Holocaust had not hit.

I knew for awhile that something was wrong. He struggled to remember the simplest of words. He was irritable. His sense of smell was off--cinnamon smelled like paint to him. I showed him almost every day how to retrieve voicemail on his phone--but he still couldn't remember.

Who thinks that someone who's not yet even old enough to retire could be suffering from a form of dementia? I didn't. Even his long-time family doctor didn't. Stress. High blood pressure. Maybe a little depression over preparing to close the chapter on his working career. We were willing to blame it on anything--except what it really was.

By the time we realized what was happening, I was so paralyzed with anger, despair, fear, and grief that I could hardly function. I went through the motions of caregiving, generally dead inside. I poured what was left of my heart out on paper:

The Hikers
by Donna StClair

We've hiked from here to there, my love
more places than I can tell.
We've hiked the Devil's Corkscrew
and down to the Ranch as well.

We've climbed the Columbia River Gorge
and Smith Rock where I almost fell.
Clear across Scotland, we walked the Way
to the Highlands and to the dell.

At Glacier, we climbed to Iceberg Lake;
"Hey, Bear!" was our talisman yell.
Here at home, we've trekked the Trail
where chestnuts rose and fell.

We've hiked up top and down below,
more places than I can tell.
But who could ever know, my love,
that we'd hike straight into Hell?

We're stumbling right through flames, my love
with no respite and no bell.
Who would've thought our well-worn soles
would be plodding this maze through Hell?

I do not see the end in sight
I do not hear the knell
But I know for sure what lies ahead
on this long through-hike through Hell.

Most of all, I missed my partner. All day, every day, I yearned to have meaningful contact with my best friend. He was slipping. More and more, he was becoming the child, the patient. More and more, I was becoming the parent, the caregiver. Make that heartbroken, barely functioning caregiver.

I can't give a date or event that caused me to change my thinking. I just realized that, given that I was trudging through Hell--I could choose to have the journey be either meaningless or meaningful.

I chose the latter.

So, I started putting my shoulder to the wheel in terms of fighting against dementia. I read and studied every good book and blog I could find. I found household accommodations that made life easier for him and for me. I uncovered ways of communicating that helped resolve both of our frustrations. I kept us involved socially. Overall, I thought I was doing pretty well--

Then, I realized I had been losing The Prescription Game. Not just losing--I was being whipped to a bloody pulp. The more I investigated, the more I realized that others were probably getting whipped as well. Since you're reading this, I'm willing to bet that you believe you might be part of that sad group of losers.

Not anymore.

INTRODUCTION

Do you ever walk away from the pharmacy counter wondering how much longer you are going to be able to afford to live?

I know that feeling all too well. I have felt it more times that I can explain, choking back tears as I clutched that white pharmacy bag and rushed to my car. How much longer, I wondered, would I be able to finance my husband's expensive medications? While I might have been willing to go without for myself, I wasn't willing to make that same decision on his behalf. He deserved to have the prescriptions needed to make his life easier, and I was determined to do whatever I could to make sure that he got them.

You see, for the past several years, my husband has waged a brave battle against early-onset dementia. This has involved taking two expensive brand name medications: Namenda XR and the Exelon patch. As unlucky as he has been in contracting this unrelenting, horrible disease, he did experience a bit of luck in terms of his good response to these medications. Only about half of dementia patients benefit from these drugs. The other, unlucky half either experience no benefit or actually get worse.

Some luck, I guess, because once a patient responds positively to a combination treatment of Namenda and Aricept or Exelon, staying on that combo for life is the name of your loved one's game. If you dare to take them off of those drugs, their cognitive abilities will plummet. Worse still, re-starting the medications doesn't yield a rebound. In short, if you determine that you can no longer afford Namenda and Aricept or Exelon, you essentially sentence your loved one to a remaining life of painfully compromised abilities. Stories abound in assisted living and memory care facilities about the aftermath of those sad decisions: "She was able to dress herself and talk just fine the other day--and now, look at her!"

What a gut-wrenching choice to make. While I have no experience in medications required to treat other fatal or life-threatening illnesses, I suspect that their story is similar: you can either pay your grocery and utility bills ... or you can pay for the medications to preserve your life. Some choice.

For the lucky who are wealthy enough to pay their own way, this problem does not exist. While Nancy Reagan and Sandra Day O'Connor share my same heartbreak in having watched their capable, cherished husbands regress to the state of helpless children, these wives, at least, were spared the anguish of trying to figure a financial path to solvency. That anguish is my constant companion.

In the case of prescription medications, the wealthy can pay their own way, whatever the price. The poorest among us sometimes benefit from some form of public assistance (provided that they know where to go and what questions to ask--another book in itself). But it is we middle class Americans who have just a little too much to qualify for Medicaid or any other drug manufacturer's subsidy program. We are the ones who are left to pay bills that often are way too high, using funds that generally are way too low.

This is a tough path that we middle-class caregivers walk.

I must admit that I am so often overwhelmed with responsibilities that I generally am not able to take the time to analyze finances as I should. Most times, I give a perfunctory glance at what appears to be a standard bill-- then dash off to mow the grass, check the fluids in the car, trim the shrubs, take my husband to his day program, vacuum the house, empty the dishwasher, make the weekly shopping list, change the furnace filters, wash the laundry, clean the gutters, feed the cats, refill the prescriptions, pay the bills, return a package to the post office, put gas in the car, make dinner, compose the minutes for the HOA meeting, read the newspaper to my husband ….

So, I can't quite explain *that day*. I don't know why I looked so carefully at that one "Part D" drug chart from Piedmont Community Healthcare, my husband's Medicare PPO. And there it was: $368.64 for a 90-day mail-order prescription of Fluoxetine, a generic form of Prozac. I remembered back when our family doctor had first prescribed it for his depression and anxiety. When the doctor saw the dark look of concern cross my face, he smiled: "Don't worry, it's generic--it's cheap!"

Sometime back, I had received a mailing from Piedmont Community Healthcare, heralding the use of their partner prescription service, CVS/Caremark. "Save up to 40%" on your prescriptions, the marketing materials promised.

And so, I drank the Kool--Aid. I moved all of my husband's prescriptions from my local CVS pharmacy to their 90-day mail order service. My clue phone should have begun to ring when I had to call over and over and over again to get my husband's prescriptions in the hopper. No, they had not received the faxed prescriptions from my husband's doctor.

No, they had not received the credit card authorization for the expenditures. No, they had not received word that any of my husband's prescriptions were "processing" within their facility. No ... no ... no ...

And so it was, after the long-awaited arrival of the money-saving 90-day prescriptions, that I looked at the report from his PPO: Fluoxetine Tab 20 mg. ... "Plan Paid" $198.51 and I paid an additional $368.64 out of my own pocket.

How was that possible?

This generic "cheap" antidepressant that our doctor had reassured me about was now costing a whopping total of $567.15 for a 90-day supply.

Generics are supposed to be the inexpensive ones, I thought to myself. I began reflecting on the discount generic programs offered by Wal-Mart, Costco, and Target. Each offers a long list of medications, generally for $4 per month, or $10 for three months. Surely, I thought to myself, there must be a generic antidepressant that would be suitable for my husband's condition. A phone call might save us some money for next time. I printed out Wal-Mart's generic listing, just to see what was shown under the "Mental Health" category.

I could hardly believe my eyes! There--printed right on Wal-Mart's listing--was the exact same 90-day drug for $10 that I had just received for $368.64 out of pocket.

Even as I write that sentence today, the fact of it is disgusting to me. How can anyone claim that a price difference like that is anything less than gouging? Worse still, upon further investigation, I realized that drug companies can charge you whatever they darned well please, without penalty. Almost half of the states in our country have anti-scalping laws for music concerts, but no such protection for prescription pricing, at least none that I can find.

In short, you and I face a sad situation: some legal protection is available if someone charges us too much for a ticket to see Garth Brooks or the Rolling Stones. But if we get charged too much for the medication needed to keep us alive--there's not much recourse.

How can this be possible?

Part of the problem lies with our current lack of legitimate investigative reporting within our media and publications. When I first discovered this huge discrepancy in pricing of a generic medication, I wrote and emailed multiple outlets in the hope of forcing a spotlight on this injustice. I contacted local and national media, AARP, *Consumer Reports*, *People's Pharmacy*, *The Clark Howard Show*, *The Doctor Oz Show*, etc. To this date, I have never heard a response. I do realize that many of these entities have often reported on problems with drug affordability, but none have ever addressed this unique and troubling situation: the exact same generic drug costing $567.15 from one provider ... and $10 from another. How can anyone even read that sentence and not be outraged?

While our news outlets are so busy keeping up with the Kardashians or determining whether black lives matter as much as white lives do, our pharmaceutical industry has answered the issues of our day in a tidy fashion. Unless you are as rich as the Kardashians, you are going to face one hell of a time trying to finance the medications you need to stay alive. And they will gouge you no matter what color you are. White lives don't matter. Black lives don't matter. What matters is green money.

Nor can we simply sit back as helpless victims in a system that rapes us at our most vulnerable. That's the problem: we don't care about what's going on until our own lives are on the line--and then it's too late. It's easy enough to read about other people losing their houses, losing their savings, losing their very lives for lack of money needed to pay for necessary care. But when YOU are involved, the reality of this cruelty becomes very real, very fast.

In Ancient Athens, Solon the Lawgiver, writer of its legal code, had this to say:
" Wrongdoing can only be avoided if those who are not wronged feel the same indignation at it as those who are."

As you might imagine, I am taking time I don't have to write this little book, and it will hardly climb the charts to be on the *New York Times Bestseller List*. Nor do I have much to worry about anymore in terms of being gouged on prescriptions. Now that I know how this unconscionable system works, I know how to get around it. The cruel irony of my own situation, however, is that I am now looking at the very real likelihood of placing my husband in a memory care residential facility, where all drugs are ordered from one vendor, and I will no longer be allowed to shop around, whether I want to or not.

No, there's not much in it for me in terms of writing this book, other than to seek validity for my own life experience as a caregiver. I've made a lot of mistakes. I've failed to ask the right questions. I've learned a lot of things the hard way. But all the wisdom I have garnered counts for nothing unless someone else can be spared some of the same mistakes, some of the unanswered questions, some of the difficult lessons.

So, come along and sit down with me at the card table--and let's start playing the Prescription Game to win. I know exactly how to do it.

UNDERSTANDING THE RULES OF THE GAME

So, how does a person wind up playing the Prescription Game?

Like it or not, you wind up playing when you or someone you love takes maintenance medications in order to live.

What is a "maintenance medication"?

Simply stated, a maintenance medication is a prescription that you are expected to be taking for the rest of your life. Unlike the temporary medications that your doctor might prescribe to treat the flu or a toothache, maintenance meds generally go on forever and ever. These medications are used to treat chronic, ongoing conditions such as diabetes, high blood pressure, heart disease, thyroid disorders, dementia, arthritis, and so on. Every once in a rare while, someone can eliminate a maintenance medication for something like diabetes or high blood pressure by losing a significant amount of weight, but generally speaking, once you're on, you're on. Forever.

It doesn't take a rocket scientist to figure that these maintenance meds are the life's blood of the pharmaceutical industry. It's hard to predict profit on how many folks might wind up with the flu or a toothache. On the other hand, it's easy enough to count the numbers of patients with heart disease, diabetes, etc. Maintenance meds are the meat and potatoes of the pharmaceutical companies' diet. And--their stockholders would rather enjoy filet mignon and La Bonnette potatoes than ground chuck and spuds.

What this means is that stockholders depend on their pharmaceutical companies to develop new drugs that will yield maximum profits. That's not intended as a statement of condemnation; indeed, all of us who own 401(k) plans or other stock investments are generally invested in this very industry. We are looking to make money from this system as well. Making money is not a dirty word.

Saving lives isn't a dirty word, either. It can certainly be argued that many of us are still on this planet because of the work of the pharmaceutical industry. "Better living through science" has been our quest since the 1950s, and the drug makers have been important players. Diseases that once put people into early graves are now manageable because of the work of the pharmaceutical researchers.

That's a good thing.

It's also an expensive thing. Research and development by pharmaceutical scientists costs a lot of money. More often than not, their efforts fail. All of that work in the laboratory, all of those clinical trials, all of that investment has to be recouped somehow. Those costs are passed along to the consumers--that's you and me.

Understandable. Also understandable is the protected 20-year patent period when the work of those scientists actually yields a beneficial drug. It's hard to quarrel with that. When a company has spent bundles of money developing a drug, it certainly has every right to recoup its original investment and make a nice profit for its stockholders.

During this time of patent protection, the drug is known as a "branded" formulation. Pharmaceutical companies love this time of patent protection. They want it to never end! The reason is simple: when their drug's patent expires, so do those nice profits. Their drug will become generic--meaning that any company can reproduce it and sell it for a much lower cost.

 But, while pharmaceutical companies love their brand name medicines, Insurance companies hate them. They don't want to pay those high prices on your behalf. They want you to pay the price. The same is true of Medicare; once they have spent over the yearly allocation of what they determine to be a reasonable investment in your prescription care, they want you to pay the price. It's called "the donut hole." And once you fall into it, everyone but you is getting fat.

Generally, you wind up in the hole once your total year-to-date drug costs reach $2,960. From that point--until you have paid $4,700 out of your own pocket--you will pay 45 percent of the negotiated price of brand name drugs. Generics will cost you 65 percent.

Whether private insurance or Medicare, expensive brand name drugs will be in an upper "tier," which is short for high priced. Insurance companies, also eyeing their own profits, don't want to pay the whole price for expensive brand name medicines. They are itching for the brands to become generic. Once that happens, they usually create a pricing structure that will encourage you to go for the cheaper kind.

From a business standpoint, all of this makes financial sense. The problem is this: it makes no ethical sense. Patients on maintenance medications--that's people like you and me--wind up caught in a tug of war between pharmaceutical companies that want to make maximum profits and insurance companies that don't want to pay into that pot on your behalf. That tug of war rips and tears at your pocketbook at a time when you can least afford to pay the price.

And the worst is yet to come: drug companies, hating to see their patent period dry up, often start hawking variations to extend their brand. It's the old "new and improved" marketing scheme. A three-times-per-day drug is introduced in a branded "extended release" formulation that you only have to take once a day. "What a convenience for your elderly patients who might be inclined to forget their drugs," the pharmaceutical rep explains to your doctor. Your doctor, who is thinking more about your health than your wallet, might be likely to prescribe that new drug for you.

Ditto for transdermal patches and all other improvements that may or may not actually increase your health. But one thing is certain: they do decrease your wealth.

By now, many consumers know to ask for generics when available. Many physicians prescribe generics when possible. But the Prescription Game doesn't end there.

Here's a little known trump card that the drug companies hide under the table: you can wind up paying hundreds of dollars more for the exact same *generic* medication in a slightly different form.

That's how I lost the Prescription Game the first time I played. I didn't just lose. I pretty much got the stuffings kicked out of me.

A COUPLE OF CHARTS TO PONDER:

Profitability of Pharmaceutical Manufacturers Compared to Other Industries, 1995-2007

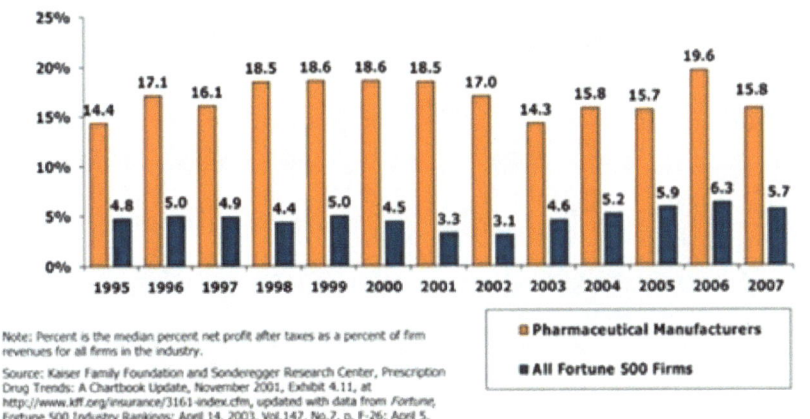

Note: Percent is the median percent net profit after taxes as a percent of firm revenues for all firms in the industry.

Source: Kaiser Family Foundation and Sonderegger Research Center, Prescription Drug Trends: A Chartbook Update, November 2001, Exhibit 4.11, at http://www.kff.org/insurance/3161-index.cfm, updated with data from *Fortune*, Fortune 500 Industry Rankings: April 14, 2003, Vol.147, No.7, p. F-26; April 5, 2004, Vol. 149, No.7, p. F-26; April 18, 2005, Vol. 151, No.8, p. F-28; April 17, 2006, Vol.153, No.7, p. F-26; April 30, 2007, Vol.155, No.8, p. F-32; 2007 number from Fortune 500 online and personal communication.

☐ **Pharmaceutical Manufacturers**

■ **All Fortune 500 Firms**

If you are inclined to feel sorry for the pharmaceutical folks who so often cite the high investments they make in research and development, take a look at this profitability chart, from the Kaiser Family Foundation. How much more profit could they expect?

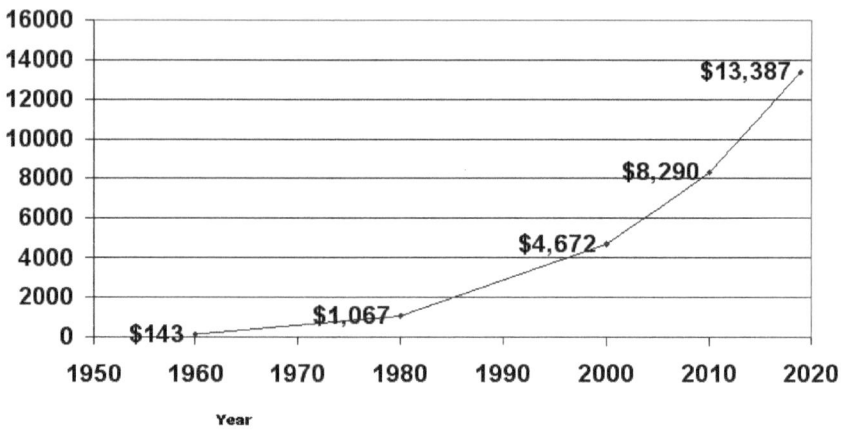

Annual U.S. Healthcare Expenses per Person by Year

Source: http://www1.cms.gov/NationalHealthExpendData/downloads/proj2009.pdf

Source:DeVoe J, Dodoo M, Phillips RJ, Green L. Who will have health insurance in the year 2025? Robert Graham Center [online].

On the other hand, take a look at our escalating healthcare expenses. The price of health is climbing higher and higher. Soon, health will be a commodity for the wealthy and the lucky.

22

HOW I LOST MY ASSets

A few years back, I accepted the fact that my husband's prescription medications were going to present a real challenge to our monthly income. Because he was battling "early onset dementia," meaning that he was diagnosed before he was 65-year-old, he was not eligible for Medicare when he first was approved for Social Security Disability. (What most people don't realize is that those younger folks who are approved for disability don't quality for Medicare until 28 long months after the fact. Given that most people who qualify for disability can no longer work, I'm not sure what our government expects them to do to afford their needed medications during this time.)

I worked for a while longer, hoping to stretch out our health insurance for as long as I could. Eventually, of course, I had to retire early, knocking the wind out of my planned retirement funds. There was just no way I could afford to work and pay someone to care for my husband. Those numbers did not compute.

So, I took early retirement. For many years, we had planned for our "golden years" by living frugally and retiring debt free. We were in a better spot than many others. What we had amassed as our nest egg, however, was intended for a songbird. What we wound up with was an albatross.

Pinching every penny became a way of life. I shopped for my clothes at Goodwill. I went back to my old newly-wed trick of making three meals out of one chicken. I turned the AC up and the heater down. Every expenditure was examined under the microscope. Every one, that is, except for his prescriptions. He was responding well to the combination of

Namenda XR and the Exelon 24-hour patch; no way I was going to mess with success.

Once he finally qualified for Medicare, I breathed a sigh of relief--at least, until I found out the meaning of the "donut hole." Basically, because he was taking expensive brand name medications, Medicare was only paying for a sizeable portion for the first five month of each year. After that point, he fell into the hole, meaning that I was paying a big chunk of it out on my own pocket. Ouch.

Through those years, whenever his doctor had prescribed medications for his dementia or depression or high blood pressure, he had always asked: "Which pharmacy should I phone this to?" I had always replied, "CVS, Cottontown"--the store almost within walking distance of our home. The kind folks who work there were always courteous, helpful, and responsive. I did and still do think the world of them.

I never thought to price our drugs around. My husband was taking two brand name meds and two generics. I thought the price was going to be pretty much the same from place to place. Little did I know.

When I received a marketing promotion from his Medicare PPO, Piedmont Healthcare, heralding the prescription service from their 90-mail mail order partner, CVS/Caremark, I was overjoyed. "Save up to 40% on your prescriptions," the materials read. I bit.

I should have known from the start that the impersonal service of a mail order system was not going to be helpful for me. My doctor's office had to fax the prescriptions three times before they were finally received and acknowledged.

During that time, I ran short on one of his medications and had to dash up the street for an emergency seven-day supply until the 90-day bottle could get through the mail.

I made phone call after phone call trying to get the paperwork straight with CVS/Caremark. No, they couldn't take a copy of my Durable Power of Attorney for my husband electronically; I had to submit a paper copy via mail. No, they hadn't received that POA yet; they couldn't talk to me about my husband's medications because of HIPAA privacy laws. No, they couldn't process out his medications yet because I had not authorized my credit card to be charged...

You would have thought I might have heeded the warning signs by now, but no. That promise of savings was ringing too loudly in my ears to hear anything else.

So, the medications finally came, and the VISA card was charged, and I had a fleeting feeling of just a smidgen of success.

Before I explain what went wronger than wrong with this service, let me first say a few things about U.S. mail order prescription services in general:

If you plan to use one of these services, understand that you will be charged for the entire 90-day supply from the moment your order processes out from the facility. In short, you own those medications even before they hit your mailbox. Nor will you be able to return them in the event that you stop taking the meds, have a different medication prescribed, or even if you die. You cannot return any 90-day mail order prescription medications unless they arrive damaged in transit or unless the mail order company has made a mistake. Read that again carefully. If your doctor has made a mistake in writing the prescription, that is something the two of you will have to settle independently; the mail order drug company bears no responsibility.

You might be able to figure your way through all of this if you have eyesight and patience good enough to read the dozen or so pages of 8-point legalese that arrive just in advance of your first prescription. But nobody does that, of course. The company is simply covering its backside, preparing to make a nice profit from the many things that you probably do not understand. If knowledge is power, ignorance is profit--at least, where an ignorant consumer is concerned.

And ignorant I surely was. I just assumed that I had saved us some much-needed income. So imagine my surprise when I looked at the Part D explanation from Piedmont Community Healthcare:

Namenda XR--Piedmont paid $44.65; StClair paid $401.79, and Medicare Coverage Gap chipped in $446.44. Not too bad ...

Exelon Patch--Piedmont paid $23.39; StClair paid $563.05, and Medicare Coverage Gap chipped in $624.51. About like expected ...

Generic Losartan--Piedmont paid $16.40; StClair paid $30.44, and Medicare Coverage Gap chipped in zero. Okay, that doesn't hurt too bad ...

But then came the killer:

Generic Fluoxetine--Piedmont paid $198.51; StClair paid $368.64, and Medicare Coverage Gap chipped in zero. That wasn't bad; that was god-awful.

I still remember looking at that line item again and again and again, determined that I must be reading something wrong. I even went on the CVS/Caremark website to double-check the charges. Yep, I was reading it right.

My eyesight was also working flawlessly when I checked on the websites for the generic drugs at Target and Wal-Mart. There it was in black-and-white: a 90-day prescription of fluoxetine costs just $10.

TEN DOLLARS.

At this point, I was the one who needed high blood pressure medication. If I have ever been madder in my life, I cannot recall the time. I wrote to my legislators. I used social media. I contacted consumer organizations. I sent certified letters to the CEOs of both Piedmont Healthcare and CVS/Caremark. I penned this letter to the editor which was published in the July 29, 2015, edition of the *Lynchburg News*:

> Dear Editor:
>
> If I pay $100 for a new pair of Nike tennis shoes and you get the exact same pair for just $50, then I guess I can lick my wounds and practice being a better shopper next time. But what if the product isn't shoes. What if it's insulin? Or an anti-depressant? Or high blood pressure pills?
>
> A few months ago, Piedmont Community Healthcare and CVS/Caremark sent us a mailing, heralding our opportunity to save money by switching to their 90-day mail-order

service. My husband, who has younger-onset Alzheimer's disease, takes a bevy of very expensive medicines. Obviously, I was delighted with the chance to save some much-needed money.

Imagine my surprise upon carefully examining the paperwork from my first order. CVS/Caremark had charged us $368.64 for a 90-day prescription of the generic fluoxetine. The same amount of the exact same generic drug costs just $10 from Wal-Mart and Target.

Okay, I got taken. I'll know better next time. I can figure my way around the system so that my husband's needs are met and we remain solvent. But what about those who can't?

How can we allow such a system to continue? It's one thing to let a "buyer beware" economic system function when you're looking to buy tennis shoes. But it is quite something else when someone's very life is on the line.

Let the buyer beware? Really? Is this who we are as a nation? We have a health care system that preys on the sick, the elderly, the vulnerable. Someday, you or someone you love will be in that very category.

And here's one last thing to ponder: CVS recently bought Target's pharmacies. Will Target's generic fluoxetine price soar to $368.64 ... or will CVS/Caremark's price plummet to $10. I'm betting I already know the answer to that question.

The response to that letter was overwhelming. People from all over town stopped me on the street to share similar stories and thank me for my efforts in making the situation public. Many others messaged me on Facebook. In short order, I realized that I had clearly touched a nerve.

The first call I got was from a CVS retail pharmacist who let me know that the Wal-Mart and Target $10 formulations for fluoxetine were "capsules," and because my doctor had written the prescription for tablets, that was what had to be dispensed. She also let me know that Wal-Mart's 90-day price for the same generic tablet was over $500.

"Well, then shame on all of you," I said disgustedly. "I really don't care if the medication comes in suppository form as long as it is what my husband needs and I can afford it."

Really? A price difference like that between generic *tablets* and generic *capsules*? Who is kidding whom here?

Worst of all, the pharmacist went on to explain that my doctor had probably prescribed the tablets because my husband had swallowing difficulty. In the first place, he does not. In the second place, capsules are widely considered to be easier to swallow than tablets.

So, here's a pharmacist who does not understand the brokenness of the system in which she is attempting to operate.

The insurance providers are equally clueless. A few days later, I got a call from a woman at Piedmont Healthcare who explained very nicely that I had paid this high price because I was in the donut hole. Really? I'm in the donut hole, so I have to bend over and assume the position? I could have paid $10 out of pocket, but I'm supposed to pay $368.64

instead? Again, who is kidding whom? Part of the reason I've wound up in this hateful hole concerns that fact that I'm paying a king's ransom for medications I could have bought for cheap. Equally ridiculous, this foolish company failed to realize that they shelled out $198.51 for this generic medication when they could have paid zero.

Here is an insurance provider who does not understand the brokenness of the system in which she is attempting to operate.

Finally, I got a call from CVS/Caremark corporate office in San Antonio, a nice young woman who was the manager of customer something-or-the-other. I gave her a piece of my mind. She listened kindly, then assured me that she could certainly appreciate how I felt and that I was under no obligation to do business with her company, that I could shop my prescription medications around.

"I won't, and I will," I said, marveling that I had finally found someone who would, at least, be honest about the brokenness of the system in which she operates.

You've heard the old saying: "If it ain't broke, don't fix it"? Well, this is broke, but I don't think anyone can fix it. All we can do is play the game--and play it smart.

TIME TO START THE PRESCRIPTION GAME

If you are losing the prescription game for yourself or someone you love, here's the first thing to do: Open up your medicine cabinet and pull out every single bottle you own. Make a list, using either a computer spreadsheet or good ol' pencil and paper.

What is the medicine's name?
Who prescribed it?
What is the dosage?
How many refills remain?
Which pharmacy filled the prescription?
Do you still actually take it (be honest)?

Be sure to write down every single detail about every single medication. Then--make a print-out of the generic price list from Wal-Mart, Target, Costco--anybody else you can think of. (If you lack a printer, you can stop by those pharmacies and ask for a copy.) If you have a laptop or tablet computer, this would be a good time to take that along as well. Questions might pop up between you and your doctor that could be answered handily with information found online.

With all this in hand, make an appointment with your family doctor for a "medication review." Some people take pills prescribed by an array of doctors. In some cases, these medications may no longer be necessary or may, in fact, be harmful when combined. Ask your family doctor to review the spreadsheet you created--and be ready to ask these key questions:

- Do I still need this medication?

- Are there lifestyle changes that I could make to eliminate this medication?
- Is a cheaper generic now available? (This is where your printed lists will come in handy!)
- Can I split the pill? In other words, could a double dose be prescribed at a lesser cost--and then cut in half?
- Are there alternative formulations of this medicine that might save me money--and could I use those (meaning capsules instead of tablets or vice versa)?
- Do you have any physician samples that I could have?
- Do you know of any coupons or special programs that the drug manufacturer offers for these drugs?
- Is there anything on the horizon for a similar, brand name drug that might be cheaper? (If this is the case, you'll want prescriptions for a 30-day supply instead of 90. Don't buy a bunch of expensive pills if something cheaper is just around the corner.)

Keep in mind that your doctor wants you to have the right medications at a price that you can afford. Also keep in mind that your doctor is focused on the practice of medicine--not on the particulars of the pharmacy. In other words, your doctor may not know that a particular generic capsule is significantly cheaper than the generic tablet (nor should he or she be expected to know that). Point is, your doctor wants you to be well. That's the whole reason he or she entered the field of medicine. But here's the problem: new drugs are often forefront in your doctor's mind because those are the drugs that have been heralded most recently by pharmaceutical reps. Like most people, doctors are prone to the lure of "newer is better." Be sure your doctor understands your financial limitations.

From the beginning, I have kept a list of all of my husband's medications in the "cloud," using an android app called "Evernote." With this handy compilation, I am able to share his medication list via email, social media, fax, or any other means you can imagine. Best of all, I only need Internet access to be able to sign onto my Evernote account to access his medications. Truly, a lifesaver.

Part of the success in playing this Prescription Game involves being the advocate for yourself or your loved one. YOU have to know what's going on before you can win this game.

Most important:
Never stop taking a maintenance medication that has been prescribed for you unless your doctor tells you to stop. If you can't afford the medication, check with resources at your state's Agency on Aging for help. Contact the drug manufacturer and explain your situation. In most cases, some interim arrangements can be worked out so that you can get the medicine you require at a price you can afford-- at least, until something more permanent can be worked out between you and your doctor.

STEP ONE: "I'LL TAKE PAPER, PLEASE!"

"Where should I phone in this prescription?" doctors always ask. Historically, I suppose, it was a logical question. Now, it is a terrible question.

When your doctor asks you that question, smile and say: "I'll take paper, please."

He or she is going to look at you like you have two heads. This is not what almost all patients say. Most patients have a "neighborhood" pharmacy. They use that one. It's been that way since--well, forever.

Again, probably a good idea way back when. Not a good idea today.

The variation in price for prescriptions can be enormous-- and if you don't shop around, you don't know. While this can make a difference even with your one-time prescriptions, the difference for your maintenance meds can amount to hundreds, perhaps even thousands of dollars over the course of a year.

If your doctor phones in your prescription to your habitual pharmacy, you are stuck with that, at least for the first filling. You won't have a chance to shop it around until you "transfer" the prescription somewhere else. Better to avoid that cumbersome step and shop it around to begin with.

Sadly, too many people don't realize that it is their right to shop their prescriptions from place to place. During the course of my own social media campaign about this issue, one of my husband's family members quipped: "Your insurance company tells you where you have to go to get your prescriptions filled."

Absolutely not.

In the case of my husband's PPO, Piedmont Community Healthcare, I had a choice: I could either use their system and pay $368.64 out of pocket for his generic fluoxetine --or I could write my $10 check to either Target or Wal-Mart.

Which one would you have done?

The problem is, not enough people understand that they have the right to do that. You don't have to shop where your insurance company tells you to go. You can tell your insurance company where to go and shop where you will. The real irony is this: sometimes you will pay a cheaper price out of your own pocket than by depending on your insurance company or Medicare.

That's messed up, isn't it? But it is also 100 percent true.

So, get that written prescription in your hand. Scan it and save it to the cloud (or make Xerox copies if you want to do it that way). Now--get ready for the next step in the Prescription Game: we're going shopping!

SHOPPING THE SMART WAY:
MOVE YOUR GAME PIECE ALL OVER THE BOARD!

[If you are not computer savvy, don't let this section overwhelm you. Please skip to page 42. I'll show you ways to get someone to teach you how to do this--or do it for you (free, too!)]

By now, I'm sure you have figured out that you have to be the healthcare advocate for yourself or your loved one. This takes time, energy, and know-how--three things that you, as caregiver, are likely to be short on. So, keep reading and I'll show you how to streamline the game and make short cuts all over the place.

Yes, you could simply make a list of the phone numbers of local pharmacies and start calling for prices. I use the phone sometimes myself, but there are faster ways.

Start by Googling your prescription name. Find their official website and check it out. Sometimes they might be offering a coupon or special promotion. At the time of this writing, for example, Namenda XR offered a coupon for a 30-day trial. Every little bit helps.

Generally speaking, the best coupons will come from your doctor or the drug manufacturer. Dozens of "coupon" sites exist on the Internet, but many are actually come-on's to get you enrolled in something you might not even be interested in--or to get your email bombarded with spam. Others are simply useless, not accepted by your insurer or by any of the federal programs like Medicare or Medicaid. *Consumer Reports* wisely recommends that we "avoid imitations" in the realm of prescription coupons. Good advice, for the most part.

The three current exceptions are LowestMed.com, WeRx.com, and, my favorite, GoodRx.com. All offer both full websites and mobile apps for your iPhone or Android. I tend to prefer the full websites because they are more functional and provide a ton of information. Let's go through some examples using the 20 mg. fluoxetine that was the subject of my prescription gouging.

If I had gone shopping right away at LowestMed.com, here's what I would have found about fluoxetine at my area pharmacies:

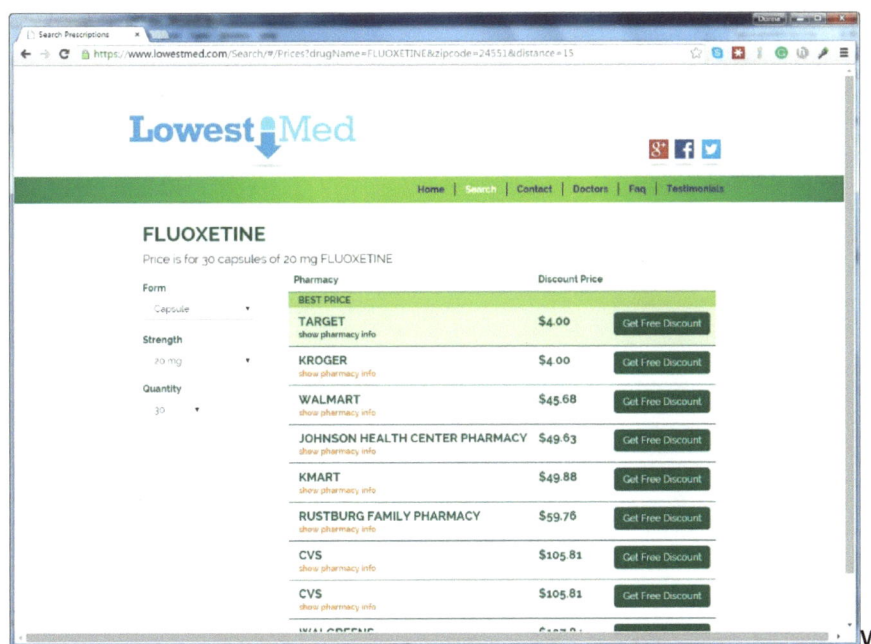

Note that this site only shows the "capsule" form. Target and Kroger reflect that terrific $4 30-day price (which translates to $10 for a 90-day supply!). But LowestMed erroneously shows Wal-Mart charging $45.68 for fluoxetine. This isn't what Wal-Mart shows on its list of generic drugs. That's why you need to check multiple sites, including the source site as ell. Keep in mind that most sources, like Wal-Mart, have both fully functional websites and smartphone apps, so that you can check prices on the go.

Another useful website with smartphone app is WeRx.com (http://werx.org). Here's what popped up when I searched for my fluoxetine:

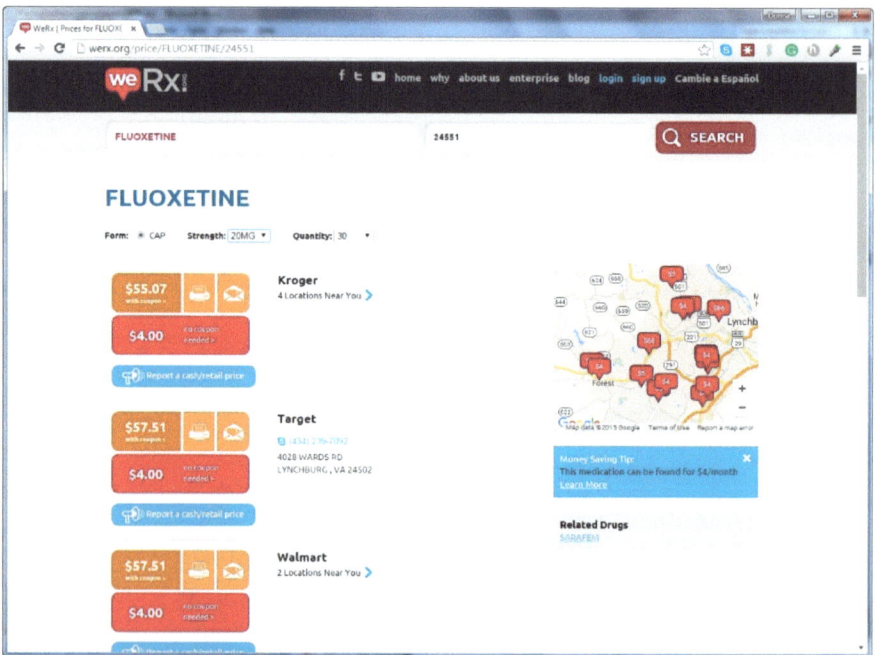

At first glance, I might have been discouraged at the pricing-- and the only option is for the "cap" form. But take a closer look at the red button below that price, and you'll see that blessed $4 for the generic capsule. Hoorah!

Again, you'll want to visit the source's website for confirmation (or make a good old-fashioned phone call). But this looks pretty promising, doesn't it? Big savings on the exact same medication--in a capsule instead of a tablet.

Next, let's look at my favorite go-to site, chock full of all kinds of drug information.

When you go to GoodRx's website (http://www.goodrx.com/), you will find a homepage that explains their process for finding the lowest prices and discounts for every FDA-approved prescription drug at more than 70,000 U.S. pharmacies. (That's more phone calls than you or I could make in a lifetime.) You are also given a search option right from that page to check on your particular medication.

When I typed in "fluoxetine," I was immediately taken to a comparison page that showed numerous locations for the $4 generic monthly--in CAPSULE form.

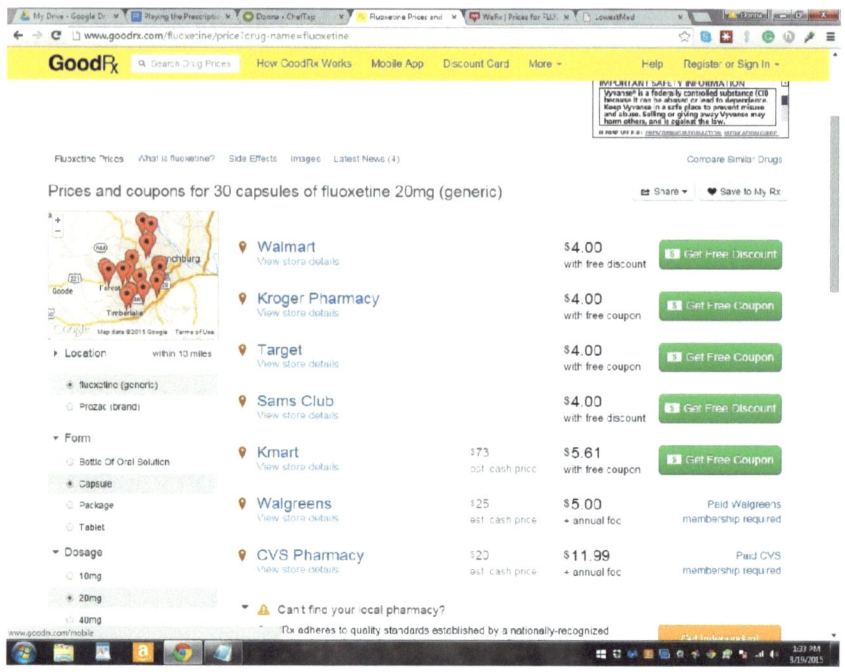

Numerous buttons on the left sidebar, permit changes in form (capsules, tablets, etc.), dosage, and quantity of pills. Really very handy! Across the menu at the top is helpful drug information--including side effects, even detailed pictures of the pills so that you will know that you've gotten the right drug. Also there is a "latest news" button. You can check there to see if there is something you should know about the drug you are taking. They even provide access to "similar drugs" to see how the price of what you are taking stacks up against comparable medications.

But when I change the form option to "tablets," here's the result:

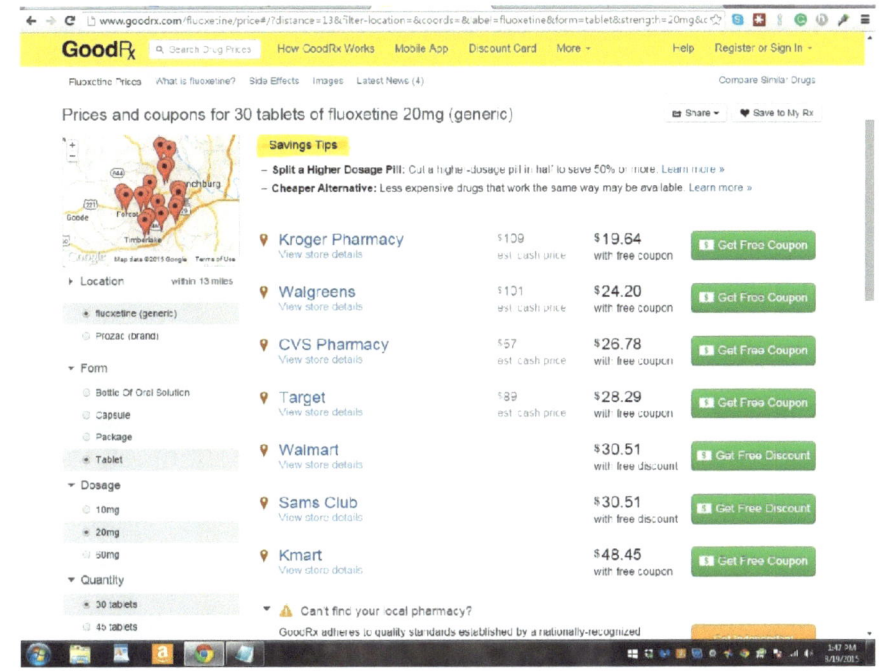

Different, huh? CVS/Caremark isn't the only offender. Seems that everyone in this game wants to charge us significantly higher prices for a tablet instead of a capsule. Why? Who knows. The only possible explanation is that the tablet could possibly be cut in half, but that's not going to cut your cost in half--so who would want to do that? Capsules are generally considered easier to swallow as well.

So here's the proof: shopping around is the key to winning this game.

Another useful feature for GoodRx is the ability to add specific prescriptions to check continuously for pricing changes. You can also add your specific Medicare plan to see how drug pricing is shaping up for you. Very helpful!

NO GOOD WITH A COMPUTER?
--YES, YOU CAN STILL PLAY THE GAME!

If you aren't computer literate, I hope you didn't even read the previous chapter because I'm sure you are mightily discouraged. Don't be. (And if you are computer literate, don't waste your time reading this part. Skip ahead.)

I'll bet you dollars to donuts that there is a young person in your family, your church, or your neighborhood who is a true computer geek. They abound everywhere. Best of all, they like doing this kind of stuff. It truly is a "game" to them.

If you can afford it, think about sweetening the pot by offering your young computer geek your first month's drug savings as an incentive to the game. Do that--and wait and see how hard he or she will work to save every single penny for you. It'll be a beautiful thing to watch.

If you can't afford such an incentive, remember that there are lots of programs out there encouraging young people to do good things as volunteers. Check with local churches. Check with local schools (the high school where I used to teach actually has a "community service" requirement for graduation; a project like this would certainly fulfill needed hours.) Check with Girl Scout and Boy Scout troops. Maybe a badge can be earned with this kind of work.

The point is this: many young people are genuinely desirous of showcasing their abilities--and if they can do a good turn in the process, so much the better.

Ask for help--and you're probably going to be amazed at how many offers you get.

You might even float your need by your local library or area Agency on Aging. They could, in fact, sponsor an event with computers and volunteers ready to do the work for you and other community participants.

And finally, once you've gotten your prescriptions straight and pocketbook back in order, I encourage you to take advantage of the many free or low-cost courses for beginning computer users. You'll find them at your local library, community college, senior center, etc. Dive in and get started, and you'll wonder how you ever survived without these skills.

Once you've gotten savvy, pay it forward by volunteering to show others what you know.

PLAYING THE GAME: COLORING OUTSIDE THE LINES

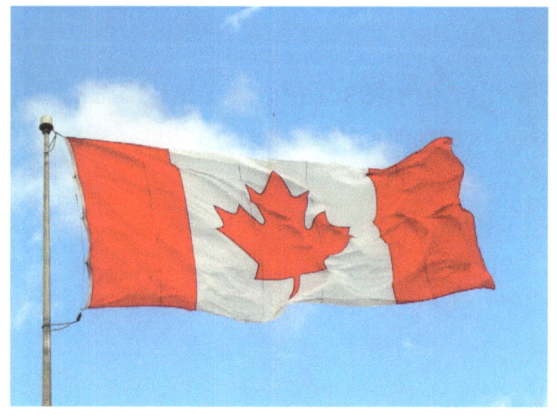

Now that you see how much money can be saved in the U.S.--just wait until you check out what's going on up north.

"Oh Canada--With glowing hearts we see thee rise, The True North strong and free!"

Yes, Virginia, there is a Canada--and they have pharmacies and reputable prescriptions just like us. Imagine that! Some 5 million Americans are already buying their drugs from our great neighbor to the north. I am one of them.

Despite the drug companies' best lobbying efforts to ban the purchase of foreign prescriptions, our government hasn't succumbed to their pressure. Yet.

Right now, the official policy of the U.S. government is that, while the purchase of non-domestic prescriptions is technically not legal, a regular consumer like you and me can buy up to 90-day's worth of a non-narcotic prescription medication for our own use--and no one will bother with us. No handcuffs. No arrest record.

In other words, our government has promised simply to look the other way. (As many complex problems as we face, I am somewhat heartened by the fact that our government has decided not to go after sick people who are just trying to find affordable medications. It's hard to understand what could be criminal about that.)

Before I start waxing poetic about Canadian pharmacies, let me give you the caveats:

- TAXES
  Any monies that you spend abroad on prescription medications will not be tax-deductible.
- MEDICARE/PRIVATE INSURANCE
  Any monies that you spend abroad on prescription medications will not add up toward getting you out of the "donut hole" and your U.S. insurance will not be accepted
- FRAUD
  Any monies that you spend abroad on prescription medications could wind up thrown down a rat hole-- and there's no one to help you. Yes, you have to be careful. There are people out there in Internet-land waiting to take advantage of you. (But we've already seen how that's possible with drug companies in our own country, haven't we?)

Take a look at those first two bullets--taxes and Medicare. Generally speaking, you will often be able to thumb your nose at these concerns because you will come out way ahead by purchasing your own medications strictly out of your own pocket.

The last bullet is the source of many people's worst fear: fraud. How on earth can you know which websites are those from genuine, reputable Canadian pharmacies--and which are the handiwork of thugs who sell sugar pills out of their basements?

Actually, it's easier than you may think. All you need to do is conduct your drug search through PharmacyChecker.com-- and then look for this symbol at any website to which you are directed:

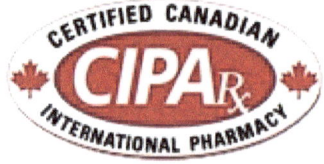

This is essentially a double form of protection that means your Canadian pharmacy requires a valid prescription, keeps your personal health profile to avoid problematic drug interactions, employs a licensed pharmacist on staff to supervise all dispensing, ensures your privacy and confidentiality, and forbids the sale of controlled substances or narcotics.

Could a mistake be made? Of course. Drug mistakes are made in U.S. pharmacies all day, every day. According to the 2006 report "Preventing Medication Errors" from the *Institute of Medicine*, "medication errors" injure 1.5 million Americans each year and cost $3.5 billion in lost productivity, wages, and additional medical expenses. Thinking that any other country operates error-free would be ludicrous. Mistakes are made.

Whether drug shopping in the U.S. or Canada or anywhere else--how can you safeguard the health of yourself or your loved one? Obviously, you want to know the name of the drug you are taking. Check that name on the label. If the drug is a refill, check that a pill from the new bottle looks like a pill from the old one. If you have questions, go to GoodRx.com and check for a photograph of the pill in question. As always, BE YOUR OWN ADVOCATE.

In the case of some Canadian pills, you will not be able to search for a confirming photograph online as easily as you can for American pills. Not to worry. If you have any questions or concerns about a first-time filing from a first-time pharmacy, simply take a pill to your local compounding pharmacist and ask him or her to verify its identity. This may cost you a little, but your peace of mind is worth it.

Be smart, be alert, ask questions--and you will have no problem doing business with a reputable Canadian pharmacy. And that's the exact same good advice for doing business with a reputable American pharmacy.

THE GAME IS NOT THE ONLY GAME IN TOWN

Looking around for the best prices on LowestMed.com, GoodRx, and WeRx can give you a real feeling of power as a consumer. But just wait until you get to PharmacyChecker.com. You'll feel like the winning ninja warrior of the Prescription Game.

The United States is not the only game in town.

Some years ago, when retirees on fixed incomes first started floating the idea of prescription shopping in Canada, the drug industry lobbyists came out swinging.

"No, we can't have that! Consumers won't know what they're getting."
"How will we even know what drugs are being dispensed."
"They aren't regulated by the same rules that we are."

 You would have thought that our Canadian friends lived in a third world country and mixed medicines up in their bathtubs. Balderdash.

Initially, the AARP supported Canadian purchasing as a viable option for seniors with expensive prescription needs. Now, however, they have their own prescription drug plan, operated by a company called Catamaran. That was a little disappointing, frankly. It's hard not to see the conflict of interest when an organization that is supposed to be advocating on behalf of saving money for seniors winds up with its hands in their pockets as well. While this AARP drug plan is a freebie with membership, one can only wonder what percentage of Catamaran's sales go into the AARP pot. Thanks all the same--I'll take Canada.

Our trip up north begins with a visit to PharmacyChecker.com. It looks like this:

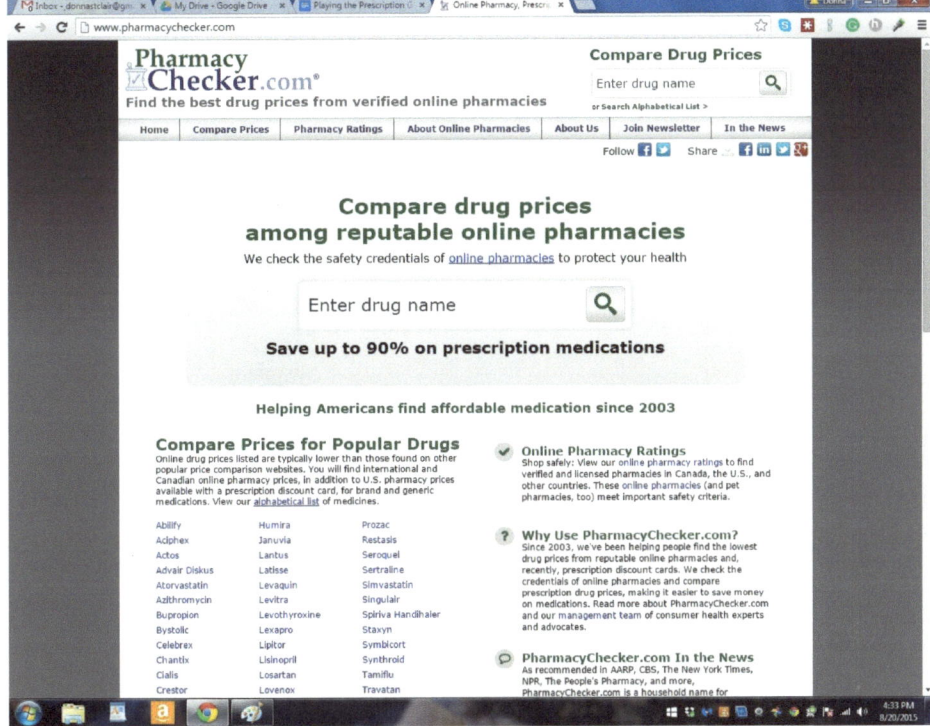

It's a cinch to operate. All you do is enter your drug name in the box as directed.

But first, let's build up to the WOW. Let's imagine that we are looking for the Exelon 24-hour patch, 9.5 mg., a drug that currently is available only as a brand name in the U.S. Let's go to LowestMed.com and see what we find:

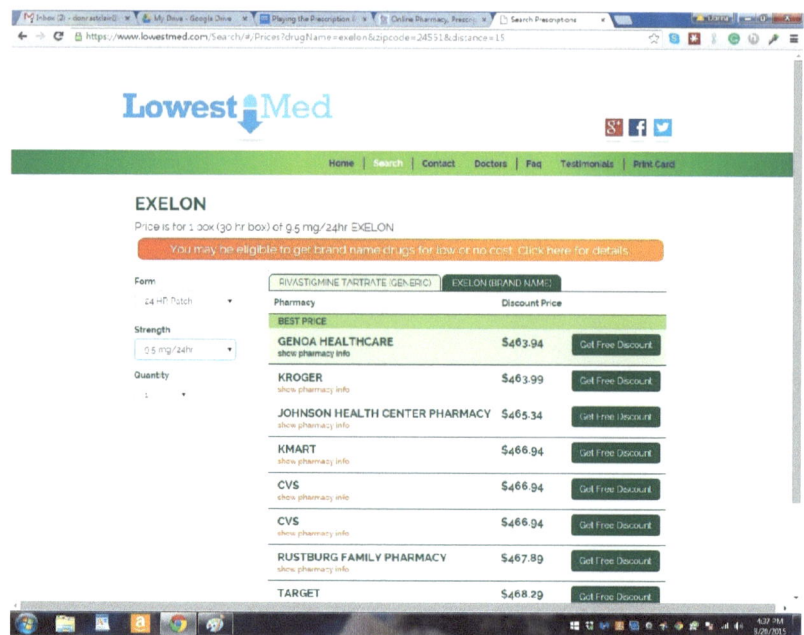

Ouch. We're talking serious money here--just for one month's worth. The numbers are about the same at GoodRx. The story at WeRx is even worse, with one month prescription running around $490. Who can afford this, month after month after month? Imagine that it's just ONE of your medications, too.

We're back to the beginning: do I want to eat and pay the electric bill … or do I want to pay for my medications?

Thank you, Canada, for showing us another way!

Here's what happens when you search for the generic patch of the exact same medication on PharmacyChecker.com:

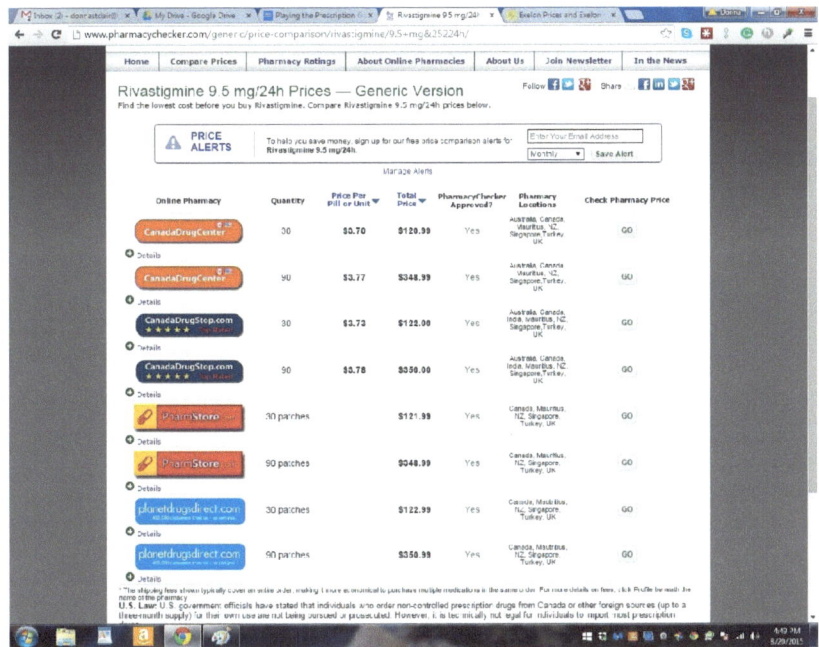

Check these 30-day prices--around $120. My heart is starting to sing "O, Canada--"! I can buy the medication that my husband needs for $120 a month there … or I can pay around $470 here. Where is the choice in that? Only a fool pays $470 for something he could get for $120. A fool … or someone who doesn't know how to play the game.

And now--you are neither of those. You know how it's done, and how to do it.

And here's more great news: most of the pharmacies on PharmacyChecker.com will match or beat the prices of other Canadian drugstores. You don't even have to shop around!

THE GAME ENDS-- AND YOU WIN!

As of this writing, here's how my husband's 90-day medication costs added up:

Losartan/HCT Tab 100-12.5 - $20.24 from Kroger
        (formerly $30.44 out of pocket from CVS/Caremark)

Exelon patch 9.5 mg. - $348.00 from PharmStore, Canada
        (formerly $562.05 out of pocket from CVS/Caremark)

Memantine HCL 30 mg. - $150.07 from Costco
        (formerly $401.79 for Namenda XR from
CVS/Caremark)

Fluoxetine 20 mg - $20 from Wal-Mart
        (formerly $368.64 from CVS/Caremark)

Pretty impressive, huh? While I once paid $1,362.92 for three-month's worth of his medications, I now pay just $538.31 -- or $179.44 per month. We can almost take a weekend trip to the beach on the savings! Your savings could be ever higher, depending on which drugs you take. Just remember this simple formula:

1. Review ALL medications with your doctor.
2. Ask for paper prescriptions that specify "substitution permissible."
3. Shop in the U.S., using LowestMed, GoodRx, and WeRx.
4. Shop in Canada, using PharmacyChecker.com
5. ENJOY YOUR SAVINGS - you earned them!

AFTER THE GAME

You know, of course, that this game will never really end. As long as you keep on taking medications and the drug companies keep on making medications, this life-and-death tug-of-war is going to continue.

Obviously, your best interests are served by doing everything possible to take care of yourself or your loved one so that you don't wind up with a medicine cabinet full of drugs. As much as possible, take responsibility for your own health. If you're overweight, get busy losing those pounds, and you may well see a reduction in your medication regimen. Weight Watchers used to say that participants who lost at least 10 percent of their body weight could generally count on being able to drop at least one of their maintenance medications. That's a powerful incentive!

Because the state of your health changes over time, plan on having that medicine review with your primary care physician every year or so, just to be sure that everything you take still is necessary. For example, I recently learned that my husband has another health situation that will likely lower his blood pressure, meaning that his Losartan will probably become unnecessary in the months ahead. I am monitoring and tracking his blood pressure several times each week.

You also need to monitor the costs of your drugs: just because Costco, for example, might have been the cheapest supplier for your first order, does not mean that they will continue to be cheapest. Have you ever wondered why Kroger, K-Mart, Harris-Teeter and many other pharmacies offer such seductive incentives--free gas, free gift card, free groceries-- for "transferring" your prescriptions? It's because their marketing research has shown that once consumers start filling a maintenance medication someplace, they tend to keep on filling that maintenance medication in the same place. Profit for them; potential loss for you. So, buck the trend.

About six weeks before your 90-day prescription runs out, start checking online once again, using GoodRx, WeRx, and Lowest Med. Also, keep an eye on Canada, using PharmacyChecker.com. Most U.S. pharmacies no longer price match on prescription drugs, but Canadian pharmacies generally do. Use this to your advantage when you want to skip the trouble of moving your prescription from one to another.

And one last tip for ongoing monitoring and control of your prescriptions: If you don't yet have a Gmail account, set up one in order to create news alerts on Google for the name of each drug you take. Go here and Google will coach you through the simple steps: https://www.google.com/alerts

Basically, you put in the words of the drug in question, "losartan," for example, and then tell Google how often you want to receive news items about this topic. Then, just sit back and let Google monitor the whole Internet for you. If there is a problem with the drug--you'll be among the first to know. Same for competitors, generic status, etc. You will know more about your medications than either your doctor or your pharmacist --and that's the kind of position we need to be in as consumers. Knowledge is power.

While you're on a roll setting up Google news alerts for your prescription names, also create one more:

drug price app

Why? Right now, I can report great success with GoodRx, WeRx, LowestMed.com, and PharmacyChecker.com. But that's for today. Who knows what new comparison websites are right around the corner? This Google alert will help you keep your fingers on the pulse. One word of caution: check out any new drug app with at least two independent, reputable news sources (*Consumer Reports*, *U.S. News and World Report*, Clark Howard, broadcast network news, etc.) As I've said before, bogus sites abound on the Internet simply to grab your email address and market more stuff to you. That's the last thing a busy caregiver or sick person needs.

By now, you might be thinking that all of this seems like a lot of trouble, that surely there must be a better way to get needed medications to sick people without all of this ongoing detective work. Well, there should be. But until that day comes (which will involve a complete overhaul of our healthcare delivery system), you and I must play the game to win--because unless we do, we are the ones who lose.

Even as a write this, I just happened to check on the price of a medication that I am taking for chronic heartburn (I'm thinking the drug industry has given me that heartburn, but I don't suppose I can prove it.) I had it filled through my insurance company's 90-day mail order service, Express Scripts. Actually, I had stopped taking it (a no-no) because I couldn't afford it. Express Scripts charged me $212.85 for Lansoprozole DR Caps, 30 mg. Last night, I could hardly sleep for that awful burn. "Time to price the prescription," I said to myself this morning.

I simply Google'd it first, to see what would pop up. Well, hush my mouth--guess what popped up? Good old Amazon. Seems this drug isn't generic; the darned thing is an over-the-counter.

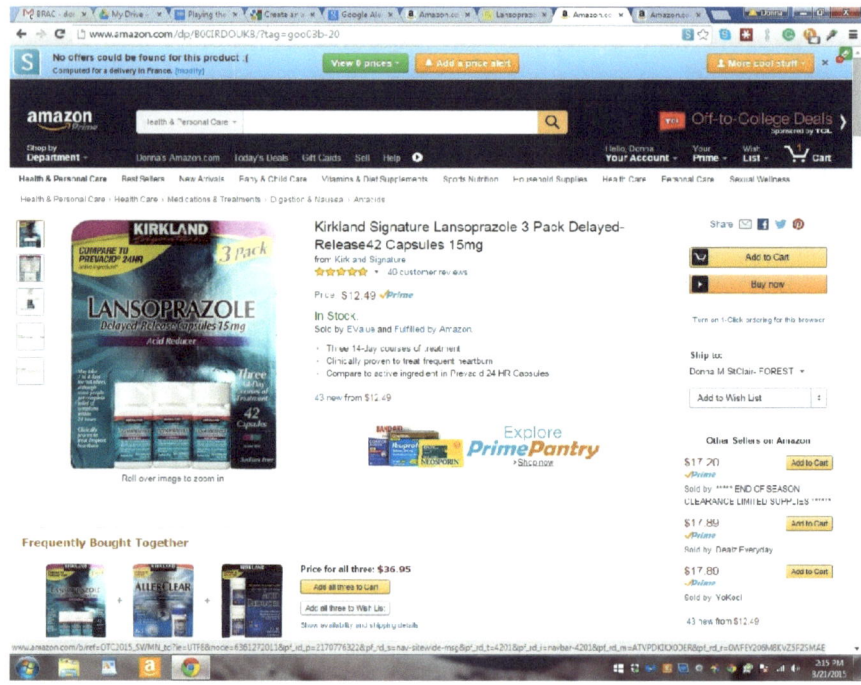

No, your eyes don't deceive you: four of these $12.49 boxes roughly approximate the prescription for which I paid a whopping $212.85.

Where does it end?

It doesn't.

That's why you and I have to keep on Playing the Prescription Game to Win!

POSTSCRIPT

Among my many initial letters, e-mails, and phone calls was one to the Office of the Attorney General of the Commonwealth of Virginia. They checked into things and received a long, rambling response from Piedmont Medicare Advantage, explaining everything that no one ever wanted to know about that infamous "donut hole."

Good ol' Piedmont provided a lengthy detailed answer--to the wrong question.

Once again, they just don't get it. They think I am upset over paying my share, now that I've fallen into that hateful hole. They just can't quite process the fact that I wouldn't even be in that hole if I were not being charged an outrageous price for a generic drug. Nor can they comprehend that they, too, have been paying an outrageous price for that same drug.

How hard is this for anyone to understand:

WHY would anyone want fluoxetine *tablets* for $368.84 when fluoxetine *capsules* are available for $10?

There is no difference. It's the same medication. In fact, if the nod goes to either form, it would be the capsules, since they are generally regarded as easier to swallow.

Now that I've finished this little booklet and gotten you on your way to winning the Prescription Game, I'm headed to Richmond, Virginia, to talk to my state senator, the Attorney General's Office, the *Richmond Times-Dispatch* …

This is just wrong--and somebody is going to listen. Stay tuned.

"Perseverance is a great element of success. If you only knock long enough at the gate, you are sure to wake up somebody."

--Henry Wadsworth Longfellow

RESOURCES

Evernote
--the tools you need to stay organized across all your devices
https://evernote.com/

Google "Alerts"
--track drug news, generics, etc.
https://www.google.com/alerts

GoodRx
--compare U.S. prices, print free coupons & save up to 80%
http://www.goodrx.com/

LowestMed
--find the lowest U.S. prices for brand name and generic prescription drugs
https://www.lowestmed.com/

PharmacyChecker
--find the best drug prices from verified online Canadian pharmacies
http://www.pharmacychecker.com/

WeRx
--help report U.S. prices and spread the word
http://werx.org/

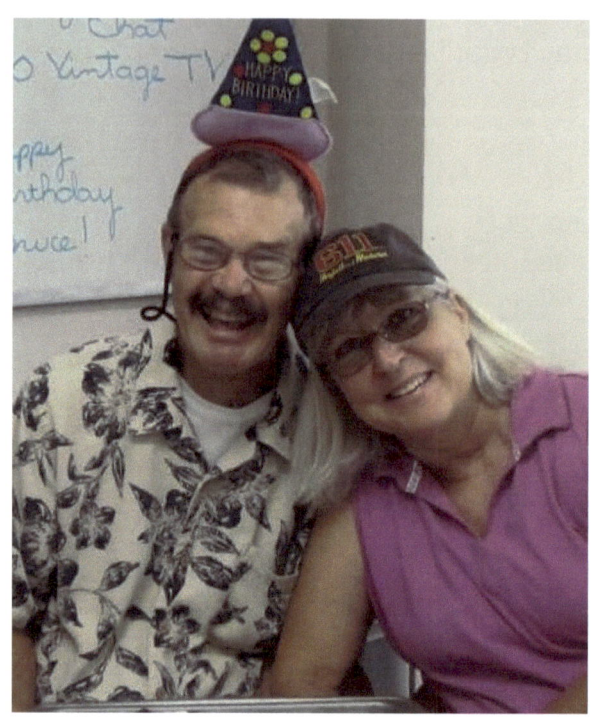

ABOUT THE AUTHOR:

Donna StClair has been married to her boyfriend, lover, dance partner, hiking buddy, and best friend for more than 40 years.

She is a U.S. Army Vietnam-era veteran who won awards in both journalism and broadcasting. Following her military stint, she earned her bachelor's degree in English and secondary education from Randolph-Macon Women's College in Lynchburg, Va. Later, she received her master's degree in communication from the University of Oklahoma in Norman, Ok.

Donna spent most of her working career in public relations and marketing, but she always said she was going back to the classroom to teach. That's what she did for the last seven years of her working life. The faculty and students at Nelson County High School hold a very special place in her heart.

She took early retirement in order to be with her husband, Bruce, after he was diagnosed with dementia. The two of them enjoy spending time with dear friends and laughing at the antics of their two cats, Lady Di and Blossom.

Donna would like to thank the staff of the Adult Care Center of Central Virginia for the wonderful care, activities, and programs that they provide for participants like her husband. All proceeds from this book are being donated to them.

She would also like to thank Sharon Celsor-Hughes and the staff of the Alzheimer's Association of Central and Western Virginia for the outstanding "Arts Fusion" music and museum opportunities that they provide for those with cognitive disabilities.

Lastly, Donna gives a big hug to her best friend, Mary Dietrich. Mary worked with Donna's husband for 13 years, during which time the three of them became like family. "I could not do this without Mary," Donna always says. The two are known most often as "Lucy and Ethel" for their adventures and misadventures in yard and house maintenance.

You are welcome to contact Donna with your comments or questions: prescriptiongame@gmail.com

www.ingramcontent.com/pod-product-compliance
Lightning Source LLC
Chambersburg PA
CBHW040325010626
45792CB00024B/2123